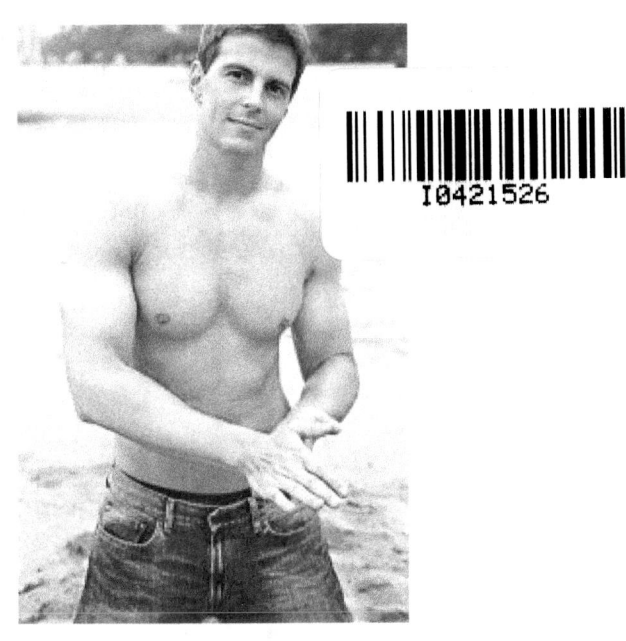

Master Healthy Living Now

10 Rules That Give You Maximum Health Today!

Published By Shaharm Publications

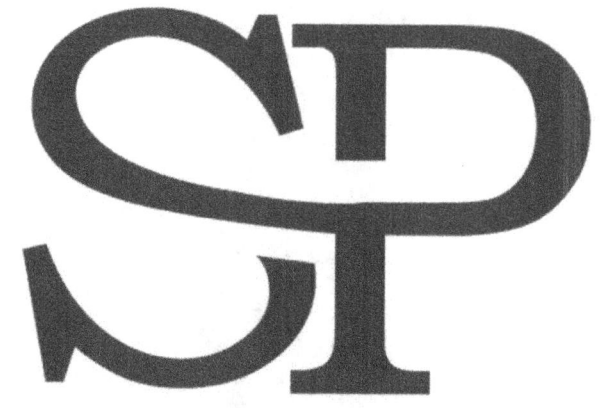

SHAHARM PUBLICATIONS

For a full list of books by Shaharm Publications, please go to:

http://www.shaharmpublications.com

Table of Contents

1. Time to Live a Healthy Life

All of us have a desire to live a healthy life and if you are currently not living the life that you want, this publication can assist you. It makes it very easy for you to follow the rules, step-by-step, so that you can attain a higher level of health and enjoy the benefits that it has to offer.

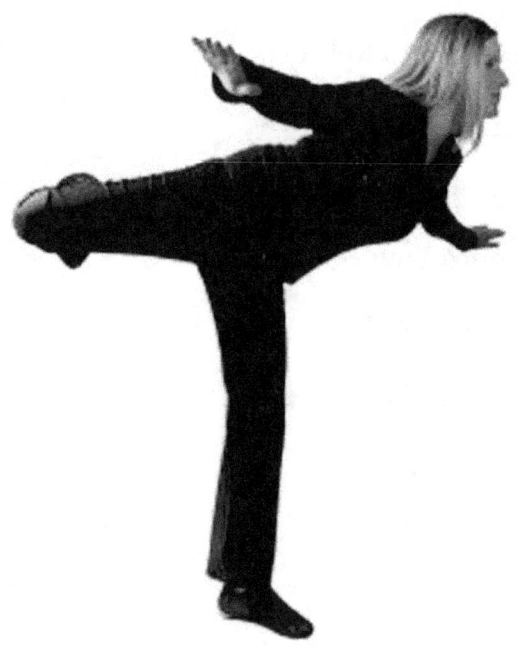

Admittedly, each of our circumstances is different and not all of us are going to be able to obtain the same level of health by following each of these individual rules. If you continue to apply them in your life, however, you will find that your health is improving and that your happiness is improving along with it. What are some of the key factors that will be reviewed in this publication?

Diet and Exercise - Well-Known Factors

The first subjects that are going to be covered in this publication are the need to get the proper diet and exercise in your life. These are factors that you likely already know and you have probably heard them many times in your life. In this publication, we are not going to review them from a generic standpoint but rather, we are going to discuss some of the best methods for improving your health through diet and exercise that have been scientifically proven.

More than likely, you have done some research on diet and exercise in the past but it may come as a surprise to you that much of the available research is flawed. It tends to be passed on from one so-called professional to another, and even though there is no sound basis for evidence that it works, it continues to be given. In addition, you will be surprised to learn the secrets behind the commercial diet companies that are not truly interested in helping you to lose weight.

Water, Water Everywhere

Another important factor that we will consider in this publication is the extreme possibility that you are dehydrated. As a matter of fact, many of us have been chronically dehydrated since we were very young and it causes a number of health issues that are very difficult to manage. In this publication, we not only discuss the amount of water that you need to drink but how you can modify the water so that it is healthier for your body.

Are you under any stress? You would be in the minority if you felt that you had no stress in your life! Many of us are dealing with a level of stress that is becoming chronic in nature and it can affect us on a very personal level, both mentally and physically. When you look at the information in this publication, you will be surprised to learn that it is not removing the stress from your life. After all, that is an unrealistic goal. What it will do, however, is help you to cope with your stress so that it does not affect you so profoundly.

When I say the word social to you, what comes to your mind? Like many people, you probably think about social media, such as Facebook, Twitter and LinkedIn. These are newcomers to the scene and, although many people measure their lives by the amount of friends they have on Facebook, it is not truly a healthy outlet. We will discuss the need to become truly social and how today's electronically connected social networks are ruining our ability to communicate.

Do you look to the future? Many people look to the future with skepticism or perhaps even with fear, but the most successful people look to the future with optimism. In the seventh role of establishing a healthy life, we are going to talk about the need to set goals and to modify your future so it works to your advantage. Although many of us may have goals, dreams and ideas about the future, very few of us write them down and pursue them. This book will change that factor in your life.

Finally, it is important to consider our connection to the world around us. No, I'm not talking about social media and getting together with friends, I'm talking about actually being connected with your environment and taking advantage of the physical items that are at our disposal. This is also something that's missing from many of our lives and it is killing us slowly, causing us to be sick and cutting short our lives in many cases because we tend to live on concrete floors with fluorescent skies.

The information that is provided in this publication can benefit anyone who wants to take advantage of it. When you begin to apply these rules in your life, you will find that you are getting healthier by the day and that you are enjoying the benefits that a healthy life has to offer.

2. Why Do You Want to Be Healthy?

When you imagine being healthier in your mind, what is it that you see? More than likely, your idea of a healthy lifestyle is much different than somebody else's idea since we are all unique individuals. It is important for you to envision it, however, and to truly see yourself attaining the goals that you now establishing. In addition, you need to be realistic in what you are pursuing, so that you are able to obtain it as well.

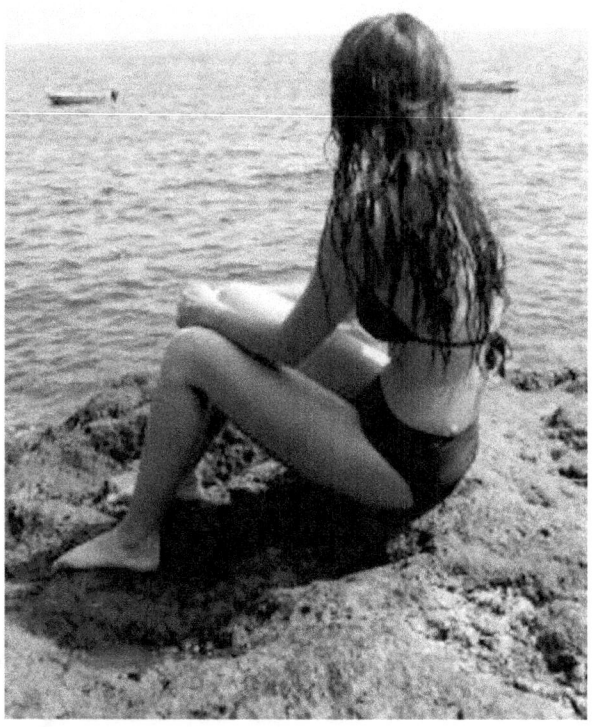

It is also important to understand that the benefits that we will receive from pursuing a healthy life are going to differ from one individual to another as well. For example, somebody that is dealing with a serious medical issue and who is trying to pursue a healthy life may just want to be healthier, even though the disease itself is incurable. On the other hand, somebody that already experiences a relative degree of health may simply want to go back to it so that they can have more energy, clarity of mind and less depression.

The purpose of this chapter is to introduce you to some of the primary benefits you will experience when you lead a healthier life. Although it certainly is true that your experiences may be different than somebody else's, these are typically benefits that we all have in common.

Energy - One of the first things that most people recognize when they begin to lead a healthier life is that they have more energy. More than likely, you have low energy throughout the day now and you may find it very difficult to get through the day without crashing in the middle of it. Once you begin to improve your health, your energy levels will improve along with it.

Clarity of Thought - Our brain makes up a very small part of our body but it uses a lot of energy. When we are unhealthy, the energy that is necessary for sustaining our thoughts is shifted to other areas of the body, such as the digestive system and the lymphatic system for detoxification. The extra energy that you have when you lead a healthy life will supply your brain with what you need and give you clarity of thought.

Happiness - Another common problem that many unhealthy people experience is depression. This can either be a simple matter of sadness or can be a much more serious clinical depression and may have many problems associated with it. When you lead a healthier life, you tend to be happier, not only with yourself but happier as an individual. It may not completely remove depression and other mental issues, but it can go a long way in helping you to cope.

Relationship - The relationships in our lives often suffer as a result of our lack of health. This is true in almost all areas of life, including our working relationships, home relationship and even our marriage. Although leading a healthy life is not going to be a cure-all that makes all of your relationships perfect, it can certainly help you to work on them in a positive manner and to move them forward.

Time - The majority of us struggle with the amount of time that we have during the day. Admittedly, we are always going to have 24 hours at our disposal, it is how we use the time that makes a difference in our perception of it. When you lead a healthier life, it is likely that you will use your time in a better manner and you will find that you have time for more important things in life, such as working on your relationships and on yourself.

Longevity - Many of the rules that lead to a healthy life can also lead to a long life as well. In fact, many centenarians have followed these basic guidelines throughout their life and they claim that it has added to their ability to live for a long time.

Immune System - One of the side benefits of leading a healthy life is the fact that your immune system is going to function more fully. This means that you will have less illness and less of a chance that you will develop a serious sickness in your lifetime. Although your immune system is never going to completely ward off all disease, boosting your immune system through eating a healthy lifestyle is a great start.

3. Rule 1: Eat the Proper Diet

One of the most important factors for leading a healthier life is eating a healthy diet. Although most people would readily admit that they understand this fact, very few of them truly understand what a healthy diet is. It is not their fault, the world is full of misinformation that is given to us by the so-called experts and through advertising, which is cleverly designed to get us to purchase a product that is not as healthy as it would appear to be. In this chapter, we will cut through those issues and discover the truth.

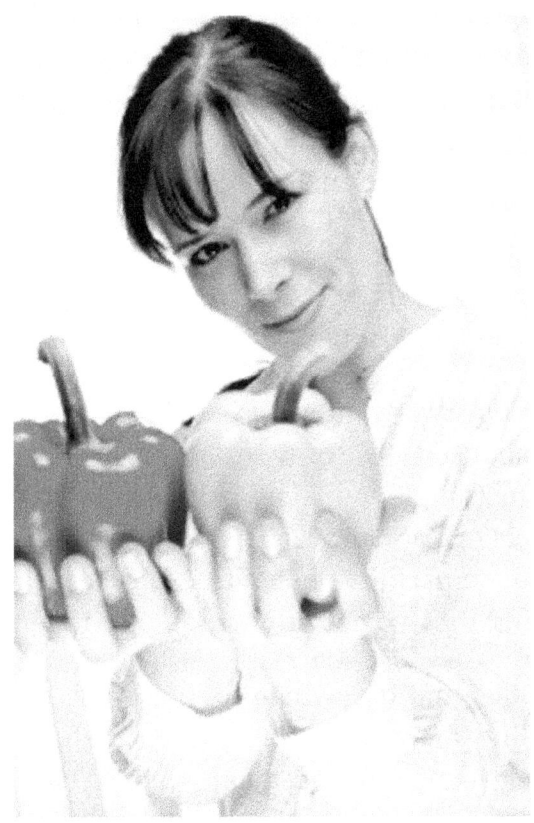

What Diets Don't Work? - Before we talk about the factors that will work for your health, it's important to understand what is not going to work. Many of the fad diets that are here today and gone tomorrow are nothing more than a quick fix and they will never be a permanent part of our life. In addition, some diets that are passed around as factual by the medical community, such as the low-fat diet and counting calories are also not truly healthy diets and they don't help you to lose weight or maintain a healthy lifestyle.

It is also important to recognize that the diet and weight loss industry, including commercial giants, such as Jenny Craig, Weight Watchers and the South Beach diet are not interested in helping you to lose weight permanently. These are commercial entities, and their primary interest is taking care of their shareholders and putting money in their pockets. If they were to teach you how to lose weight permanently, they would lose you as a customer. That is why most people who are on these commercial diets lose weight temporarily, gain it back and continue to go back for more of their products for the rest of their lives.

What Is a Healthy Diet?

The body needs something that very few of us provide for it, and that is balance. Most of the diet types that exist focus on removing something completely from our eating habits, such as low-fat diets or very low carbohydrate diets. Although these may provide temporary benefits, they are not typically sustainable and they do not provide balance in our lives.

The fact of the matter is that we need all types of foods, protein, healthy fats and carbohydrates. When eaten in the proper proportions and consistently, they can help you to maintain a slim waistline and a healthy lifestyle. Although there are many different factors that can be included in this formula, the easiest way to describe it is to eat a high-fat, low carbohydrate diet, such as the Paleolithic diet.

Of course, none of us are going to be perfect and you should never assume that you are only going to eat fruits and vegetables, meats and healthy fats for the rest of your life. From time to time, you're going to want to eat a piece of cake or perhaps go out to eat at a restaurant and not have to worry about what is on the menu. It is important for you to give yourself a treat such as this, provided it does not become a way of life that is permanent.

Dietary Secret of the Centenarians

When a number of Centenarians were polled as to why they felt they were able to live such a long life, there was one factor that was strikingly consistent in the group. It had to do with diet, but not in the types of foods that they ate, but it was when they ate and how much they ate.

Most of us that are eating the standard American diet or even those of us who may be eating a somewhat healthy diet tend to fill ourselves to the brim at every meal. Many of the Centenarians, however, said that they made it a habit to walk away from a meal while they were still slightly hungry.

It should not surprise you to learn that this is not only a secret of the centenarians, it has also been established by many health food experts, who recognize the importance of remaining hungry. No, you do not need to starve yourself but if you to shoot for about a 75% full rate on every meal, you will be heading in the right direction.

4. Rule 2: Get Some Exercise

The second rule of achieving and maintaining a healthy lifestyle is to add some exercise in the mix. Most of us will also agree that we should be getting some exercise but in today's world, which tends to promote a sedentary lifestyle, very few of us get the exercise that we need. In fact, we may even find that we are becoming breathless, simply walking upstairs to bed at night. Without the proper exercise, we are not only losing our healthy edge, we are killing ourselves.

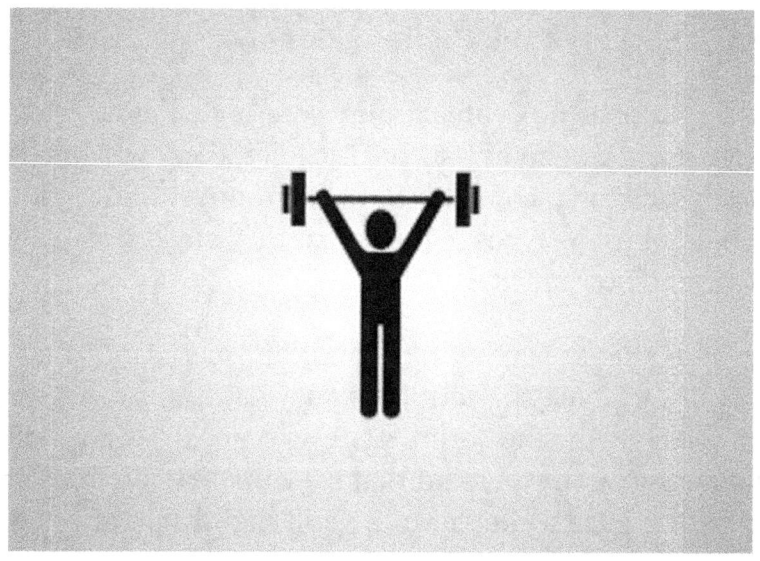

Most people's perception of exercise is somewhat skewed in comparison with the truth of what we really need to maintain our health. If your idea of exercise is going to the gym for hours a day, sweating it out with a bunch of muscle heads, grunting and groaning as you throw iron around and flex your muscles in the mirror, you are mistaken. As a matter of fact, you don't even need to join a gym to get the exercise you need and it only takes a matter of 90 minutes per week, if you exercise properly.

Two Types of Exercise Is That You Need

There are two primary forms of exercise that should be included in your weekly regime, aerobic and anaerobic. Aerobic exercise, which includes activities such as walking, running, bicycling and swimming, engages the cardiovascular system and causes you to breathe heavily. In fact, the word aerobic, which means "with air" is very descriptive of the type of exercise and the way that it makes us feel.

Anaerobic exercise, on the other hand, does not require additional oxygen to our muscles. It includes exercises such as weight lifting and certain calisthenics that can be done at home, including push-ups, pull-ups and dips. These types of exercises work the muscles and it helps to build lean muscle mass, which truly makes us a healthy individual.

You should be doing the mix of both aerobic and anaerobic exercise in your weekly schedule. If you exercise properly, in the way that we will discuss in this chapter, you don't need any more than 90 minutes of exercise per week. Most, if not all of us, could easily fit that into our schedule.

How to Exercise Properly

You will find many different ways to exercise described online and in books at your local library. In fact, you can get lost in all of the discussion and most of those forms of exercise will not only promote themselves as the best type, they will also put down any other type of exercise that goes against their methods.

In this chapter, we are going to discuss the easiest and perhaps most effective way for you to exercise both aerobically and an anaerobically. In fact, it is a combination of the two, and when you do it properly, the 90 minutes of required exercise per week may actually be too much.

Introduction to Slow and Steady Circuit Training

Have you ever watched people working out at the gym lifting weights? If you truly understand the principles of the lift, you will recognize that most people are doing it wrong. Some people tend to throw the weight around, lifting it then dropping it as quickly as possible in order to get as many reps in as they can. Other people, on the other hand, load the bar with so much weight that they are only able to do one or two repetitions.

In the slow and steady circuit training camp we are going to hit a happy medium. It involves engaging the muscles to the fullest extent possible and doing so while watching your form as closely as possible. This will allow you to get the most out of your weightlifting activity and when you do it properly, it will also provide you with the aerobic activity that you need as well.

Types of Exercises - There are hundreds of different types of exercises that can be done at the gym, all of which provide some type of benefit. For our exercises, however, we are going to focus on what is known as "multi-joint" exercises, which engage multiple muscles in the body. This allows you to work out your muscles in a shorter amount of time and to get the benefits of the exercise to a greater extent.

Some of the most common and easiest ways to do multi-joint exercises include the bench press, deadlifts, squats, Yates - bent over rows and the shoulder press. When you do these exercises in the circuit, you will work almost all of the muscles in the body and you will be able to do it in a very short amount of time.

How Much Weight to Lift? - It is also important for you to strike a balance when it comes to how much weight you are lifting. This is a number that will differ from one individual to another, but your primary goal is to maintain perfect form until you are no longer able to maintain it again, a condition known as failure. You will want to be able to do a minimum of eight repetitions with perfect form and a maximum of 12 repetitions. Once your strength increases and you are able to do more than 12 repetitions, you should increase the weight on the next session.

How to Lift - The most important factor to consider when lifting in this way is that you should follow a very strict and perfect form. Do not throw the weight, providing momentum and do not push the weight by twisting or wrenching the body that could lead to injury. Follow perfect form and once you are unable to lift the weight any longer with perfect form, you are finished with that exercise.

It is also important to consider how quickly you are lifting. During each exercise, you will have both a positive and a negative movement. Each movement should take you a full four seconds to complete. Do not rush the exercise, or you may naturally try to use momentum. By maintaining a slow and steady pace throughout the exercise, you will experience more benefits.

The Importance of Rest - Some exercise gurus will tell you it is necessary to hit the gym every day or perhaps to go a minimum of three or four times a week. That is far too much. Your muscles do not grow while you are exercising, they grow while you are resting. You should only exercise in this way two times per week, maximum. Some people even find it beneficial to exercise in this way one time per week.

By giving your body the proper rest, you will see your strength and muscle mass grow quickly. It is a very effective form of exercise, and although it may be somewhat untraditional, it works very well if you are patient enough to do it.

5. Rule 3: Learn How to Be Moderate

Throughout the pages of this publication, we are discussing many different factors that can be used to improve your health. In this chapter, we are going to talk about a role that is very important to keep in mind when trying to improve your health, the role of moderation. After all, many of us become so focused on improving our health that we can go all out and before we know it, we burn out and stop trying. In addition, we may have certain habits that need to be moderated as well. In this chapter, we are going to discuss both of those factors.

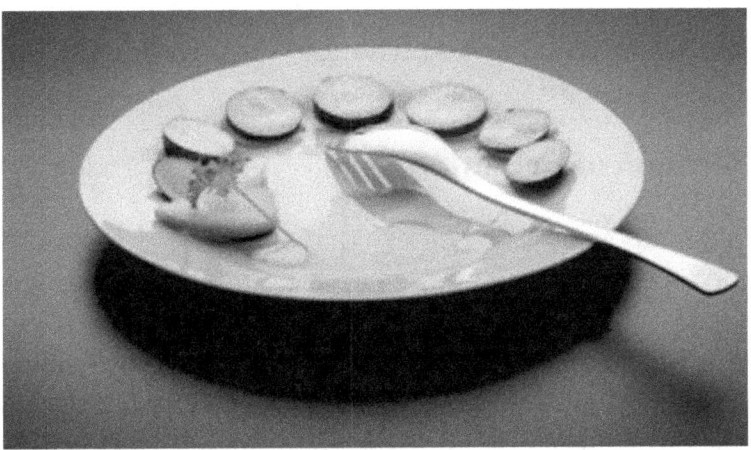

Taking a Look at Your Habits

All of us have habits and we tend to live our lives in association with those habits, which govern our conduct and how we spend our time. When you truly understand your habits, you will begin to recognize that some of them are controlling you to the point where it is causing difficulty. It is important for you to stop and to make any adjustments that are necessary through moderation.

An example of how we may need to be moderate is in our eating habits. Many of us tend to eat until we are full but this may not be the best choice if we want to lead a healthy and long life. As was discussed in rule number one on our diet, most centenarians have followed a natural regime during their lifetime where they walked away from the table, even if it was available. When you apply this type of moderation in life, you may find that you have many benefits come your way.

Another area to moderate is the amount of alcohol that you drink. Although there certainly is nothing wrong with having a drink now and then, drinking too much alcohol can damage your health and impair your senses. Moderating your consumption will allow you to enjoy this precious gift without ruining your health in the process.

Moderation or Cessation?

It is also important to recognize that some habits are unable to be moderated. In some cases, the habit has become so ingrained that it is going to be impossible for us to limit the amount that we do it. For example, many people that smoke cigarettes cannot limit how many that they smoke, the only option for them is to quit. The same is also true with many other negative habits, such as drug addiction and gambling.

If you have negative habits that you need to remove from your life entirely, you will never be able to return to it again. Just one cigarette or one ounce of gambling will generally cause you to return to your habit, because of the way that it is ingrained in your mind. If you have a habit that is not negative and you are able to moderate it, you should do so. If you must remove it from your life, however, it needs to be a permanent removal.

The Need to Seek Balance in Your Healthcare

Another form of moderation that is very important to discuss is the need to moderate your desire to seek a healthier life. When you begin to get healthier, and experience the benefits, it can cause you to obsess over your health and it can rule your life. In an effort to get healthier, you may actually be picking up some very unhealthy habits and lifestyle changes that need to be removed.

It is always best if you seek balance in your life, regardless of whether you are talking about improving your physical health, your mental health or even your emotional health and relationships. Without that balance in place, you will surely not be able to obtain the higher level of health that you desire. In fact, it may be counterproductive and you can find that you are slipping backward as a result of trying to move forward so quickly.

If you work on your health and take steps in the right direction, you will experience the benefits that we discussed at the beginning of this publication. It is important to consider it to be a progressive action, however, and not one that you are going to leap into with both feet. As long as you are making positive ground, you will continue to experience the benefits and enjoy all that a healthy life has to offer.

6. Rule 4: Adjust Your Sleeping Habits

One of the activities in life that many of us take for granted is the time that we are sleeping. In reality, we spend more time sleeping than we do in any other activity and in most cases, it overshadows those other activities by a long shot. That is why it is important for you to think about the sleep that you are getting and to recognize that it is important when it comes to your health and happiness.

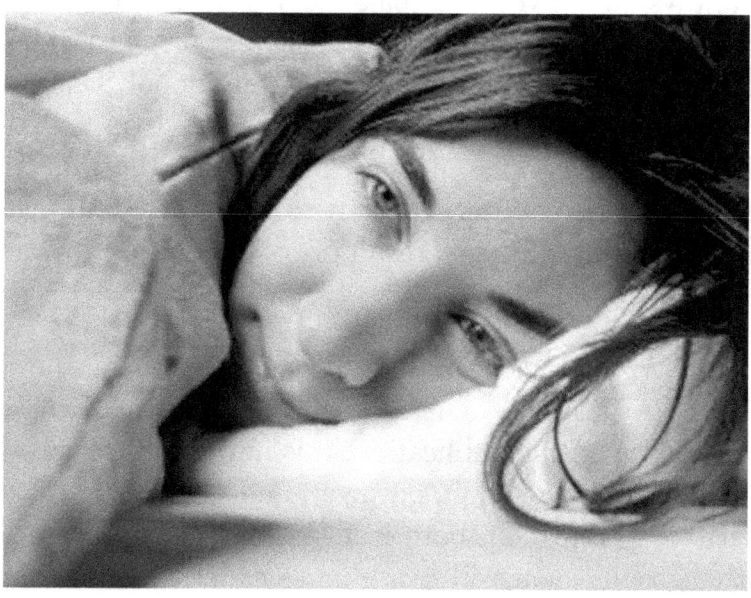

Unfortunately, many of us tend to look at sleep as being expendable. We may even find it to be inconvenient and we do everything possible to avoid sleeping and the time that is required to do so. If you are not getting enough sleep, however, you are harming your health in numerous ways. Not only will you feel sluggish and ill during the day, you are building up sleep debt and eventually, the debt is going to need to be paid.

There are many different factors associated with your sleep that could be considered in this publication. We are going to focus on just a few, however, that can help you to sleep better and to enjoy the benefits that being well rested has to offer.

Timing Your Sleep - You will read information from a variety of sources that tell you that the best choice is to wake up early in the morning and get started. "Early to bed early to rise" is their motto, but is there any truth to it?

Some people are going to function quite well in the morning and they may be able to get a lot more work done, if they wake up early and get right to it. Other people, however, are going to find that they are not firing on all cylinders in the morning and it may take them quite some time to fully wake up and get started. These individuals generally call themselves night owls, and it is important to recognize that as individuals, we may do better at night.

There are no hard and fast rules that would govern the time that you should go to bed and the time that you will wake up. It is something that you must discover for yourself and as long as you are leading a healthy and productive life, you can adjust your schedule to suit your needs.

What is important to consider is consistency when it comes to going to bed and waking up in the morning. Most of us tend to fight going to bed at night, something known as sleep procrastination and it can be a serious issue that leads to sleep debt and daytime drowsiness. We may also tend to adjust our wake-up schedule, hitting the snooze alarm multiple times during the workweek and then sleeping in on the weekend.

The healthiest way for you to sleep is to go to bed every night at the same time and wake up at the same time every morning.

Your body will become accustomed to this schedule and eventually, it will even begin to wake up immediately before it is time to wake up. It is important to maintain this sleep schedule, even during the weekend and times when you may be on vacation.

Lighting up the Night

Another issue that is becoming an increasing problem is the fact that we are exposed to light before we go to bed. We all have a natural circadian rhythm that is based on a 24-hour period and, due to exposure to light in the morning, our body releases chemicals that allow us to wake up. If we expose ourselves to the wrong type of light at night, it keeps our body from producing chemicals that cause us to fall asleep, such as melatonin.

The light that would cause this is sometimes referred to as blue light and it is very similar to the light that we are exposed to from our cell phones, tablets, computers and televisions. Many of us bask ourselves in the light of these electronic devices right up until the time that we go to bed, and then we wonder why we are not able to fall asleep.

If at all possible, avoid being exposed to this type of light for at least one hour before you go to bed. If you do need to be exposed to the light, you should wear orange tinted sunglasses to filter out the light that would affect your sleep cycle.

Serious Sleeping Problems

There are a number of serious problems that can affect our sleep and can make it difficult for us to be healthy. These would include problems with chronic insomnia and sleep apnea. In this part of the chapter, we are going to discuss sleep apnea and why it is a killer.

Sleep apnea is a problem that affects millions of people and many are unaware that they have a difficulty. It causes a person to stop breathing during the night for anywhere from a few seconds to up to a minute or longer because the muscles in the throat collapse when you relax while sleeping. As your body is deprived of oxygen, you will wake up enough to take a breath, but not enough to regain full consciousness. Some people suffer from apnea episodes throughout the night and may have hundreds of them in a single night of sleep.

The primary problem with sleep apnea is that it is robbing you of the ability to get any deep, REM sleep. That is why one of the primary symptoms of sleep apnea is daytime drowsiness. This drowsiness can be so profound that some individuals have a difficulty staying awake while driving or anytime they sit still for more than a few seconds. Sleep apnea can also raise your blood pressure and increase your risk for stroke and heart attack.

If you have sleep apnea, you do have a few options that will help you to sleep better. One of the options is to go for a sleep study and get fitted for a CPAP machine. CPAP machines force continuous air into the lungs, keeping the airways open while you sleep. You can also do sleep apnea exercises, which will strengthen the muscles in the throat that collapse while you sleep. Additional suggestions for treating sleep apnea include losing weight, avoid drinking alcohol before going to sleep and stopping smoking. You may also find some relief when you sleep on your side.

7. Rule 5: Learn How to Relax

We live in a world that tends to put us under a lot of undue stress. We may experience high levels of stress in the workplace, at home and in many other situations throughout the day. Although stress can be a helpful motivator and it is a natural part of life, the chronic stress that many of us deal with on a day-to-day basis is unhealthy for our mind and body.

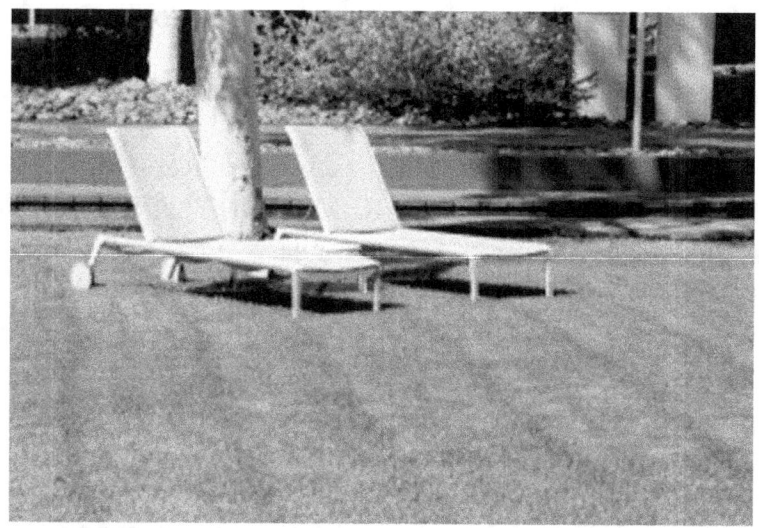

It is unrealistic to think that you are ever going to be able to completely remove stress from your life. Of course, you can remove some of the factors that are leading to stress but more than likely, it is still going to be an issue that must be considered. In this chapter, we are not going to focus on removing stress from your life but rather, we are going to discuss the method that can help you to cope with it effectively.

Deep Breathing for Stress Relief

The importance of breath in our life cannot be understated. Without our breath, we would lose consciousness within a matter of minutes and shortly thereafter, we would lose our life. Unfortunately, many of us do not breathe properly and we really only engage the upper half of the lungs. This could be because of our stress levels, which cause shallow breathing or it may be because of our posture or even a learned response.

One important factor to consider to keep yourself healthy and to reduce your stress is to focus on your breathing every day. We are going to discuss a specific breathing technique but it is also important to consciously breathe, by focusing on our breath and trying to engage the entire lungs and the diaphragm. This is something that can be done for a matter of a few minutes every day but the effects of doing it can be quite profound.

The Square Breathing Technique

If you are under a lot of stress and are having a difficult time coping with it, the square breathing technique may be able to help. This is a scientifically proven method that can adjust the oxygen and carbon dioxide levels in your body quickly and help you to relax. It can be done in any location, regardless of whether you are relaxing at home or standing in line at the supermarket. Try it once and you will be hooked, continue to use it and it will benefit you for life.

During the square breathing process, you are going to be counting to four multiple times. It is important that you do not rush this count and that you continue at the same pace throughout the process. If you ever feel stressed or have a difficulty reaching four, you can reduce your count to three but you must maintain it throughout the process.

The first step is to breathe in through your nose. You will breathe in to the count of four and fill your lungs to a comfortable capacity. Do not force too much air into your lungs. You should also make sure that your lungs are being engaged from the bottom so that you are getting a lot of oxygen. Your diaphragm should also engage, causing your stomach to move outward while you are breathing in.

During the second step of the square breathing process, you will hold your breath to the count of four. This should be a relaxing part of the exercise, but if you are having any problems, you can reduce your count to three. As you continue to use the square breathing exercise, you will become accustomed to the sensations.

After you have held your breath to the count of four, it is time to transition to the next step of the process. During the third step, you will breathe out to the count of four. Your breath should slowly and gradually escape from your lungs through your open mouth until they are comfortably empty. Do not force the lungs to go completely empty, it is fine if some air is left in them.

The final step in the square breathing process is to hold your breath while your lungs are empty. You should also count to four during this part of the exercise and it should be done in a relaxed manner. Some people find this part of the exercise to be difficult but with some practice, it will become easier.

Once you have finished the four steps of square breathing, you will repeat it three times for a total of four. It only takes a minute to do this exercise but it can be very effective at helping you to relax and to cope with stress. It is an important part of developing a healthy life.

8. Rule 6: Drink Plenty of Water

How often do you feel thirsty? If you are like most people, you are thirsty most of the time but you simply ignore the sensation. What you may not realize is that the sensation of thirst is a natural reaction of the human body to let you know that you are dehydrated. That's right... once you are thirsty, you have already gone too far and it is time to take action. If you take action and hydrate yourself properly, it can be one of the most important things you do for your health.

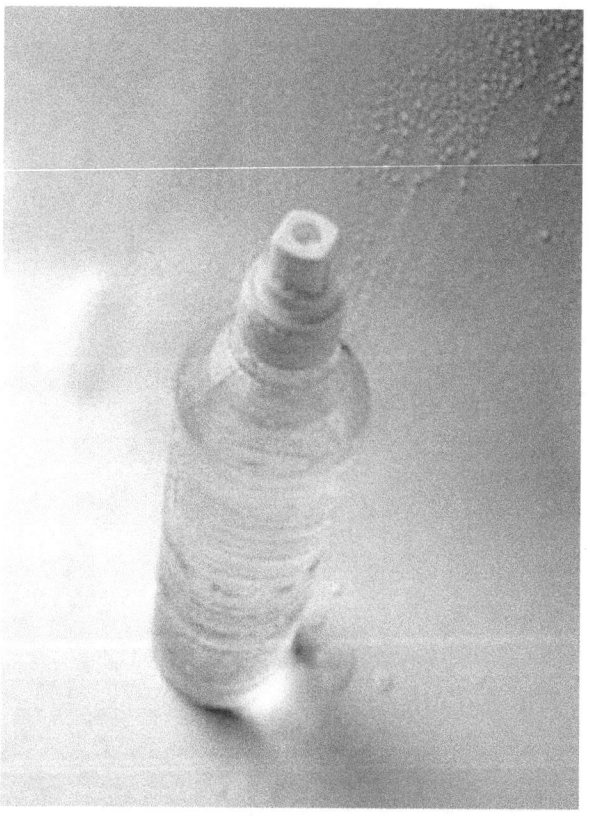

Many of us are not only dealing with a problem with occasional dehydration, we are suffering from a state of chronic dehydration. This may be something that we have dealt with for the majority of our life and it can be very damaging on the body. In fact, some experts in the natural health care field feel that dehydration is behind many of the chronic problems that we may be experiencing. Whether that is true or not, it is obvious that hydration is an important part of our health and fortunately, it is also one that is easy to correct.

How much water do you need?

One of the most common questions is in regards to the amount of water that we need to drink to stay hydrated. Most experts will recommend that you drink anywhere from 8 to 10 cups of water daily, but that may be far too low for an estimate. Of course, any amount of water that you add to your daily regime is going to benefit you, but in order to truly hydrate yourself and experience all the benefits that it offers, you need to shoot for a number that is much higher.

The easiest way for you to reach a state of super hydration is to drink half of your body weight every day in ounces of water, for example, a 200 pound man would want 100 ounces of water daily. You can adjust your drinking habits so that you are trading it in spurts throughout the day rather than drinking it all at one time.

Some people also find it beneficial to drink a large amount of water upon waking in the morning. In fact, there is a health system that is known as a kidney flush that would require that you drink a quart and a half of water within the first 10 minutes after waking up in the morning. The water should be room temperature and if you are able to do this, you will typically feel much better all day long. It also helps to knock down the amount of water that you need to drink for the rest of the day.

Another method of increasing the amount of water that you drink is to drink a full glass of water approximately 30 minutes before you eat each meal. This will also significantly cut down on the amount of water that you need to drink for the rest of the day and it aids in digestion.

What kind of water should you be drinking?

Another common question is in regards to the type of water that you should drink. Although there is a lot of information about filtered water and avoiding bottled water in plastic, those are not necessarily important factors that you will need to consider. Of course, the healthier the water that you drink, the better the benefits for your overall health but don't avoid drinking water because you don't have access to high-quality H_2O.

If the only option that you have available is to drink water out of your tap, then you should by all means do so. When possible, you can improve the quality of your water by installing a reverse osmosis water filter. Until that time, however, it is better for you to drink tap water than no water.

One other factor that you can consider for improving your water is to add some fresh squeezed lemon juice. This is not only going to improve the taste of the water, it will also adjust the pH level that is very healthy for you. It is an option that you may want to consider because it can make it easier for you to drink water and it boosts your health.

9. Rule 7: Establish and Pursue Your Goals

All of us have goals in life but not many of us are going to achieve the goals that we have set. In addition, we may have long-term and short-term goals but we never write them down and think about what is necessary in order to accomplish them. In this chapter, we are going to look at goal setting and why it is an important part of your life and your overall health.

How to Set Your Goals

There are a number of considerations for setting your goals that will make it easier for you to achieve them. First of all, you should think about both long-term and short-term goals and establish them separate from each other. Try to make your short-term goals work along with your long-term goals, so that you are working toward both at the same time.

It is also very important to write down your goals as you are establishing them. Try to keep your goals in your mind is not going to be as effective and when you write something down, it helps to establish them as something that is tangible, rather than something that is not achievable. The process of writing something down also makes you accountable to the goal as well.

How to Record Your Goals

Rather than simply writing down what you would like to accomplish in your life, it is important for you to think about the entire process. This is something that many people do not do, but it can really have an effect on your ability to pursue your goals and achieve them.

When you establish a goal by writing it down, think about every step that needs to be taken along the way so that you can maintain your focus and eventually, reach the goal. You should also look for any problems that may occur along the way and how you would be able to overcome them, if they do arise. The more information that you can put down on paper, the more likely it will be that you will stick to your plan.

Don't Forget to Review

Another aspect of goal setting that is often ignored by many people is the necessity to review your goals on a periodic basis. All of our lives are constantly changing and at times, it is necessary for us to adjust our goals according to different factors that may have come up in our life.

Although it is important for you to be diligent in going after your goals, you should not be so set in stone that you are going to ruin your possibility of achieving all that life has to offer. Continue to allow your goals to be fluid and when necessary, either adjust your course or perhaps rearrange your circumstances to meet the goal. If necessary, you could even abandon that particular goal in favor of pursuing one that is more realistic or provides you with different benefits.

Like any habit, it can take some time before setting goals and achieving them is a permanent part of your life. Perhaps you can make it your first goal, in making goal setting a part of your life and doing it every day for at least 30 days so that it can become ingrained in your mind.

10. Rule 8: Practice Your Social Skills

One important factor for our health that is often overlooked is the need to be social. For some individuals, this is a rule that is going to come naturally but for others, it will be difficult for them to put themselves in situations where they can be social. In this chapter, we are not only going to discuss the benefits of socializing, we are going to discuss the need to step outside of the new definition of what social is.

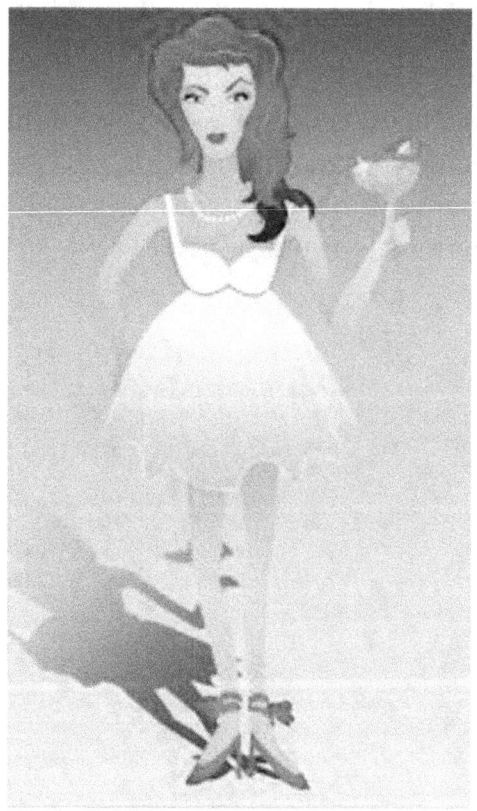

What Is Being Social?

It wasn't all that long ago that being social had a single definition, that of getting together with family or friends or being in a crowd of individuals and talking, perhaps with people that you did not know. In this modern age where we are all electronically connected, the practice of being social has changed considerably. In fact, it is ingrained with the words social media, and most of us now try to get the necessary socialization by sitting at our computers or by talking to others on our smart phones through Facebook, twitter and other social networks.

Unfortunately, we have become so electronically connected that it is now difficult for us to maintain regular social connections. If you want to see an example of what I am speaking of in action, try looking around at many of the people at a restaurant today. Although they may be sitting across the table from each other, separated by only a few feet, they are actually separated by hundreds or perhaps even thousands of miles because they are buried in their smart phones, talking to others and trying to be social in that way.

In fact, many people now measure their degree of success and their social abilities by counting how many friends they have on Facebook and the other social networks. We tend to spend more time socializing in this way than ever before, and unfortunately, it is robbing us of our ability to converse with people face-to-face.

How to Be Social Properly

The most important thing that you can do for your health as far as socializing is concerned is to detach yourself from your electronic device on a daily basis. For some people, this is going to mean putting the cell phone down on the table and actually talking to the person that is sitting across from them. In other cases, it may mean turning off all of our electronic devices and spending some time giving our brain the opportunity to reset.

There is no doubt that we need each other and the ability to be social is a skill that is becoming more and more difficult to master. If you take the time to master it, however, and form close personal bonds with individuals on a face-to-face basis, you will find that it affects your health in a positive way and it brings many other benefits that you will enjoy for a lifetime.

11. Rule 9: Ground and Sky

Our lives have certainly changed in the past several decades but some of the ways that they have changed have been so gradual that very few of us notice it. For example, in the beginning of the previous century, most people were constantly in contact with the earth. They worked in the field, and children played outside. Families gathered outdoors when the weather was nice and it seems that we spent most of our time enjoying the sunshine and the feel of grass underneath our feet.

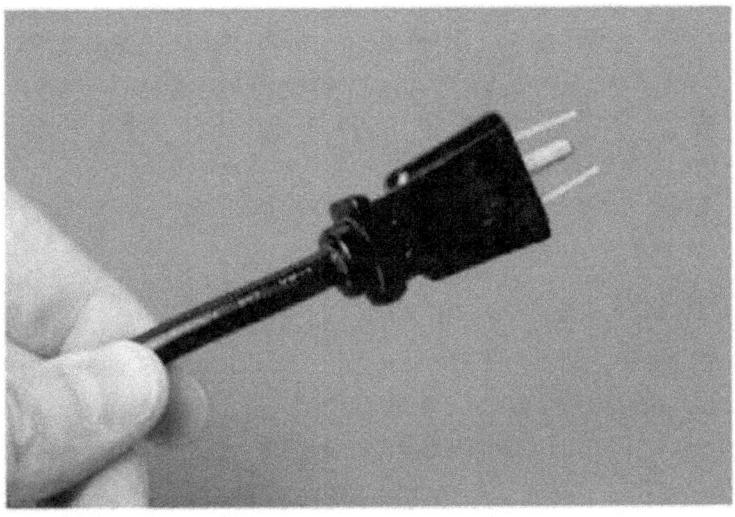

Today, things are quite different and the vast majority of us are spending our time on a concrete floor. This concrete is nowhere near as healthy for us as the true ground and to top things off, we typically live under florescent skies as well. This has had a profound effect on our health and unless we do something about it, we may find that we are hurting our health on an ongoing basis.

Of course, it is not only beneficial to be in contact with the ground because of the magnetism and energy that it provides, it can also protect us from our electronic devices as well. Although we can't see it, there is a constant electromagnetic field that is emanating from our laptops, smartphones, TVs and other electronic devices. When we are in close proximity to them, that electromagnetic field passes through us and damages us on a cellular level. What can be done to stop this problem?

In recent years, it has become more and more popular to ground yourself and avoid this difficulty. There are commercial pads available that plug into the ground of a wall outlet and when you put your feet on the grounding pad, it grounds you to it. When electromagnetic fields strikes you and you are grounded, it will not pass through you but will run along the outside of your body until it seeks ground. There are even large grounding pads that can be used on your bed so that you are grounded all night long!

Those electromagnetic fields may even be more damaging than most people realize. For example, our laptops, smartphones and tablets are often on our lap and close to our reproductive organs. There has been an increase in the amount of ovarian and testicular cancer in recent years and many specialists feel that it is the proximity of those items to that area. In addition, holding a cell phone close to your ear puts that electromagnetic field close to the area of your brain.

Ideally, we would want to remain grounded at all times but in practice, it is very difficult to do so. It is far better for you to be grounded when you are near any electromagnetic fields and if at all possible, spend some time truly grounding yourself by walking on the ground outside. Many people find it beneficial to walk barefoot in the grass in the morning before the dew evaporates. In any case, it is something that you can practice on a regular basis to provide additional health benefits in your life.

12. Rule 10: Love the Life You Live

Throughout the pages of this publication, we have discussed many factors, listed as rules, which would help to govern your life and allow you to live a life that was healthy. In this chapter, we are going to discuss a factor that many people tend to overlook, that of being content with your life and loving what you have. It is important for you to consider this, because it can make a difference in your happiness and your happiness is closely associated with your health.

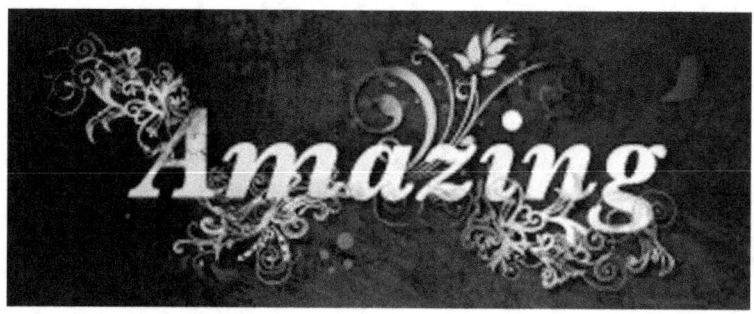

All of us have different circumstances, with some of us having an abundance of physical items and others lacking many of the items that we need on an ongoing basis. Although people exist in both forms, there is something that some of them have in common. It doesn't matter how much you have in a physical way, if you learn how to be content with what you have, it is possible to be happy.

This factor can be seen easily in individuals who have a positive attitude. More than likely, you know somebody that is positive and it seems as if they are always looking at the bright side of any situation. When an individual is positive, does it mean that nothing bad is ever going to happen in their life? That is hardly the case! As a matter of fact, many individuals who have a positive outlook on life have a number of bad things that are going on in their life at any given time. The real difference is that they are able to look beyond those negative factors and to see the positive aspects of life.

You can take a lesson from this and it certainly will make a difference in your ability to be content with what you have. There is also something else that you can do, and this can be part of your long-term goal setting. If you're unhappy with your life or with any aspect of your life that is changeable, why not do what is necessary to change it? Admittedly, some negative aspects of our life, such as serious health problems may be a permanent part of our life, but in some cases there may be aspects of our life that we can change.

Of course, making changes in our life is always going to require effort on our part and it can be difficult to put our best foot forward, when we have been struggling for quite some time. This is also somewhere that positive thinking can come in and if you can envision it in your mind and are positive that you are going to be able to achieve it, half the battle is actually won.

You really need to strike a balance in your life if you want to be content and love the life that you are living. In some cases, it may be a matter of adjusting your ideals or your goals in life to be able to love the life that you are living. In other cases, however, it may be reaching out for something better or for something that is attainable, which will make you happier with your life. As long as you are balanced and continue to be content with the things that you have, you will find that it makes you a happier person and your health will follow.

13. Healthy Living Tips

We have provided you with an abundance of information through 10 simple rules that you can apply in your life to make yourself healthy and happy. In this chapter, we are going to take it a step further and provide you with some tips that you can use in your life to maintain your health and to realize that it is well within your reach.

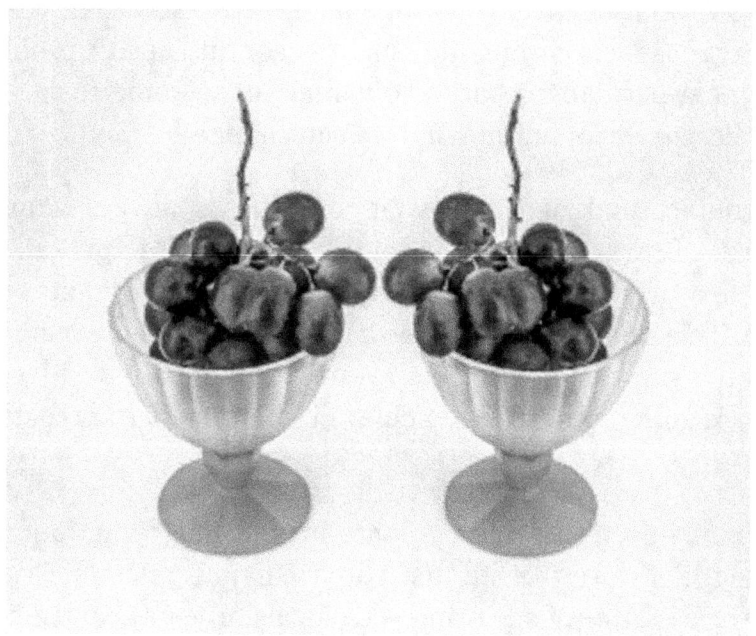

It is what you do, not who you are - Many people that are unhealthy tend to blame their problems on genetics. Although there are some instances in which genetic factors may play into our health, over 90% of all health problems are related to lifestyle choices. It is up to you to decide how you are going to live your life and the amount of health that you enjoy.

Walk Away Hungry - Although there are many factors that can make you healthy and provide a long life, a common factor among many centenarians is that they step away from the table hungry. Rather than filling themselves until they cannot eat any more, they save some room.

Drink Water - One of the most common problems that many people experience is a difficulty with dehydration. It is especially difficult as we get older and our thirst reflex diminishes. Drink enough water every day and your health will benefit.

Move - Although it is important to get regular exercise every week, it is also important to incorporate movement into your day-to-day activities. Park a little further away from the store that you are visiting or take the stairs, rather than the elevator. It will make a difference.

Smile - The simple act of smiling or better yet, laughing, can make a huge impact on your health. Take the time to smile every day.

Breathing - Don't forget the importance of breathing properly and engaging your diaphragm. It allows oxygen to enter the body and keeps you healthy. Schedule time every day to breathe.

Checkups - Although many people will want to care for their health in a natural way, it is also important for you to get regular checkups with your physician. They are not perfect, but there are times when they will identify issues that need to be addressed.

Look Forward - Many of us tend to live in the past, regretting the things that we have done or wondering how we may have changed our lives for the better. Rather than looking to the past, look to the future, because it is a part of our life that still is under our control.

Detach - When you are constantly attached to your electronic devices, they can have a very strong control over your life. Detach on a daily basis for a minimum of 10 minutes by shutting all of your electronic devices down and allowing your mind to reset.

Go Barefoot - Don't forget to spend some time outdoors, grounding yourself by allowing the feet to come in contact with the earth. The best time to do this is early in the morning before the dew evaporates.

Routine - Remember that your routine defines who you are and if you are keeping a good routine, it will contribute to your health.

Sleep - Are you getting enough sleep every night? Not only should you be sleeping enough, you should keep your sleep times consistent, including the time you go to bed and the time you wake up, each and every day.

14. Living a Healthy Life and Loving It

Although many people dream of living a healthy life, very few people are able to accomplish it. In reality, it is not a matter of wanting to do something, it is simply a matter of reaching out and taking hold of it. As we have discussed in this publication, our health is within our reach and it is a matter of what we want to do with our life and how we want to live it. In addition, we not only want to be healthy, we want to be happy and love the life that we are living.

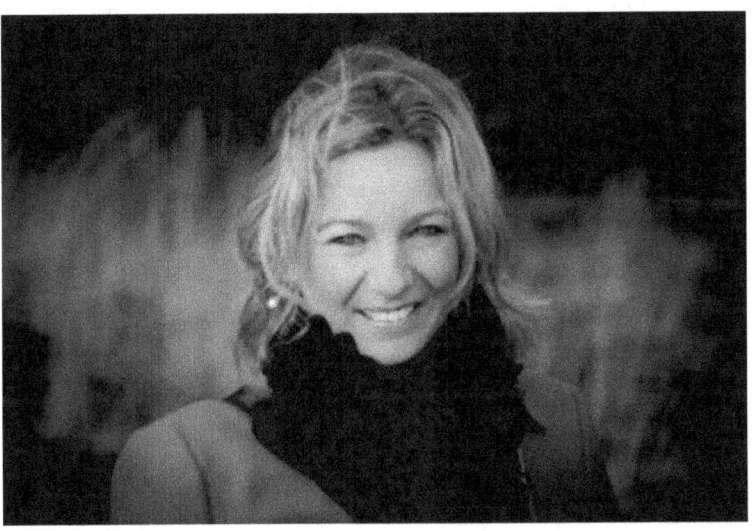

Many factors of how to live a healthy and happy life were considered in this publication. From discussing lifestyle changes, such as modifying our diet, exercise habits and drinking enough water, to setting goals and achieving them or even to grounding ourselves to the earth. All of these factors can make a difference in your life, you simply need to take advantage of what they are offering.

When you utilize the 10 simple rules that are provided in this publication, you will find that your health is improving on almost a daily basis. The benefits will begin to be experienced very quickly and as you continue to develop your life in a healthy way, they will continue to be experienced. In fact, you will likely experience many benefits that were not discussed in this publication, simply because they were specific to your circumstances.

Nobody is perfect and there is never going to be a time when we will experience perfect health, as long as we are living in our bodies as they are today. That doesn't mean, however, that we can't reach out for the brass ring and live a life that makes us happy. Take the time to incorporate the principles in this book and you will not only experience the physical benefits of living a healthy life, you will experience the emotional benefits that go right along with it.

www.ingramcontent.com/pod-product-compliance
Lightning Source LLC
Chambersburg PA
CBHW070341290526
45791CB00003B/1419